Gastroparesis Diet for Women

A Beginner's Guide to Managing Gastric Disorders, with Sample Recipes and a 7-Day Meal Plan copyright © 2022 Stephanie Hinderock

All rights reserved No part of this book may be reproduced, or stored in a retrieval system, or transmitted in any form or by any means, electronic, mechanical, photocopying, recording, or otherwise, without express written permission of the publisher.

Disclaimer

By reading this disclaimer, you are accepting the terms of the disclaimer in full. If you disagree with this disclaimer, please do not read the guide.

All of the content within this guide is provided for informational and educational purposes only, and should not be accepted as independent medical or other professional advice. The author is not a doctor, physician, nurse, mental health provider, or registered nutritionist/dietician. Therefore, using and reading this guide does not establish any form of a physician-patient relationship.

Always consult with a physician or another qualified health provider with any issues or questions you might have regarding any sort of medical condition. Do not ever disregard any qualified professional medical advice or delay seeking that advice because of anything you have read in this guide. The information in this guide is not intended to be any sort of medical advice and should not be used in lieu of any medical advice by a licensed and qualified medical professional.

The information in this guide has been compiled from a variety of known sources. However, the author cannot attest to or guarantee the accuracy of each source and thus should not be held liable for any errors or omissions.

You acknowledge that the publisher of this guide will not be held liable for any loss or damage of any kind incurred as a result of this guide or the reliance on any information provided within this guide. You acknowledge and agree that you assume all risk and responsibility for any action you undertake in response to the information in this guide.

Using this guide does not guarantee any particular result (e.g., weight loss or a cure). By reading this guide, you acknowledge that there are no guarantees to any specific outcome or results you can expect.

All product names, diet plans, or names used in this guide are for identification purposes only and are the property of their respective owners. The use of these names does not imply endorsement. All other trademarks cited herein are the property of their respective owners.

Where applicable, this guide is not intended to be a substitute for the original work of this diet plan and is, at most, a supplement to the original work for this diet plan and never a direct substitute. This guide is a personal expression of the facts of that diet plan.

Where applicable, persons shown in the cover images are stock photography models and the publisher has obtained the rights to use the images through license agreements with third-party stock image companies.

Table of Contents

Introduction	7
What Is Gastroparesis?	10
Causes of Gastroparesis	10
Symptoms of Gastroparesis	12
Diagnosing Gastroparesis	13
Medical Treatments of Gastroparesis	17
Lifestyle Changes to Manage the Gastroparesis	20
Natural Remedies for Gastroparesis	21
Gastroparesis and Women	23
What Is Gastroparesis Diet?	25
Benefits of the Gastroparesis Diet	27
Potential Drawbacks	29
5 Step-by-Step Guide to Getting Started with the Gastroparesis Diet	31
Step 1: Familiarize Yourself with Gastroparesis	31
Step 2: Shift Towards Liquid Nutrition	33
Step 3: Introduce Low-Fiber Solids Gradually	36
Step 4: Carefully Manage Fat and Fiber	38
Step 5: Keep a Detailed Food Diary	41
Foods to Include in the Gastroparesis Diet	46
Foods to Avoid in the Gastroparesis Diet	48
Sample Meal Plan for the Gastroparesis Diet	50
Coping with Gastroparesis	54
Essential Tips for Managing Gastroparesis	54
Troubleshooting the Gastroparesis Diet	56
Sample Recipes	58
Blended Soup	59
Fruit Smoothie	60
Vegetable Stir-Fry	61

Asian Zucchini Salad	62
Honey Roasted Potatoes	63
Guilt-Free Egg Salad	64
Turkey with Avocado Salad	65
Cauliflower Rice with Chicken and Broccoli	66
Lentil Soup	67
Greek Yogurt Parfait with Berries and Almonds	69
Muesli-Style Oatmeal	70
Broccoli and Cheese Omelet	71
Almond Surf Smoothie	72
Mango Honey Green Smoothie	73
Lemon-Vanilla Berry Parfaits	74
Avocado and Salmon Salad	76
Grilled Chicken Kebabs	77
Chicken Seafood Paella	79
Creamy Mashed Potatoes	81
Poached Pears in Cinnamon Syrup	82
Silken Tofu with Soy Sauce and Scallions	83
Simple Baked Apples	84
Quinoa Porridge	85
Conclusion	**86**
FAQs	**89**
References and Helpful Links	**91**

Introduction

Navigating life with gastroparesis demands patience, resilience, and a road map to manage its symptoms effectively. The condition, characterized by the stomach's inability to empty itself of food in a normal fashion, can be perplexing and often frustrating. Yet, amidst these challenges lies a beacon of hope - a carefully crafted diet tailored to ease the burdens of gastroparesis. This guide is your companion on a journey toward better health, offering insights into the dietary adjustments that can significantly improve your quality of life.

At its core, the Gastroparesis Diet Guide is about understanding the intricacies of your body and learning how to nourish it in a way that mitigates discomfort and promotes digestive wellness. The condition's nature means that standard dietary advice doesn't always apply, making it crucial to approach your meal planning with a strategy that acknowledges and respects the unique hurdles posed by gastroparesis.

For anyone grappling with this condition, the prospect of eating without fear or pain may seem out of reach. However, the truth is that with the right knowledge and adjustments, managing gastroparesis through diet is not only possible but can be a transformative experience. This guide lays down the foundational principles you need to adapt your diet, focusing on foods that facilitate easier digestion and ways to keep your nutritional intake balanced, even when your options might seem limited.

The aim here isn't just to provide a list of do's and don'ts but to empower you with the understanding and tools to make informed choices about your diet. The guide walks you through identifying foods that work best for your body, planning meals that support your digestive system, and adopting habits that contribute to a more manageable daily life with gastroparesis.

In this guide, we will talk about the following;

- What Is Gastroparesis?

Keep reading to explore how this Gastroparesis Diet Guide can become your trusted companion, regardless of where you are in your journey with this condition. It opens the door to a world rich in educational insights and adaptive strategies, each piece of advice designed to make your path through gastroparesis less daunting and more manageable. With practical recommendations and supportive guidance, this guide is your first step toward a life where food becomes a friend, not a foe, in your battle against gastroparesis.

What Is Gastroparesis?

Gastroparesis is a medical condition characterized by the stomach's inability to empty itself of food in a normal, timely manner. The term "gastroparesis" is derived from "gastro-" meaning stomach, and "-paresis" meaning partial paralysis. This delay in stomach emptying can interfere with digestion and can lead to various complications.

The condition reflects a malfunction in the spontaneous muscle movements (motility) meant to propel food through the digestive tract, specifically affecting the muscles of the stomach. Essentially, gastroparesis impairs the normal rhythmic contractions that help move food along, resulting in delayed gastric emptying without an obvious blockage or structural problem as the cause.

Causes of Gastroparesis

The causes of gastroparesis can vary, involving factors that impair the normal function of the stomach muscles or nerves controlling them. Key causes include:

- ***Diabetes***: High blood sugar levels from diabetes can damage the vagus nerve, which controls the stomach muscles, leading to gastroparesis.
- ***Surgical injury***: Operations on the stomach or the vagus nerve can damage it, potentially resulting in gastroparesis.
- ***Viral infections***: Some viral infections can lead to gastroparesis by damaging the stomach muscles or their nervous control.
- ***Medications***: Certain medications, particularly those that slow gastric emptying or affect motility, like narcotic pain relievers, can cause gastroparesis.
- ***Neurological conditions***: Disorders such as Parkinson's disease and multiple sclerosis, which affect the body's muscles and nerves, can lead to gastroparesis.
- ***Connective tissue disorders***: Conditions like scleroderma, which involve the connective tissues, can affect the stomach's lining and muscles, causing gastroparesis.
- ***Idiopathic gastroparesis***: For many individuals, the cause of gastroparesis is unknown (idiopathic), meaning it occurs without a clear, identifiable reason despite thorough investigation.

These factors can interfere with the stomach's muscle contractions, preventing it from emptying properly and leading to the symptoms and complications associated with gastroparesis.

Symptoms of Gastroparesis

The symptoms of gastroparesis can vary in severity and may include:

- *Nausea*: Feeling sick to the stomach, which can be persistent.
- *Vomiting*: Throwing up undigested food hours after eating is especially common.
- *Early satiety*: Feeling full very quickly when eating.
- *Abdominal bloating*: The stomach may feel uncomfortably full and bloated.
- *Weight loss and malnutrition*: Due to difficulty in eating enough nutrients.
- *Abdominal pain*: Discomfort or pain in the stomach area, which can vary in intensity.
- *Heartburn or GERD*: Gastroesophageal reflux disease symptoms due to the backward flow of stomach contents into the esophagus.
- *Lack of appetite*: A decreased desire to eat.

These symptoms can lead to significant discomfort and affect the quality of life, making management and treatment crucial for those with the condition.

Diagnosing Gastroparesis

Diagnosing gastroparesis involves several steps and tests to assess how well the stomach empties and to rule out other conditions that may cause similar symptoms. The process usually includes:

1. **Medical History and Physical Examination**

    A detailed evaluation begins with a healthcare provider carefully reviewing the patient's medical history, including any chronic conditions, symptoms they are experiencing, current and past medication use, as well as any surgeries they have undergone in the past. This comprehensive review is crucial for understanding the patient's overall health status.

    Following the medical history review, a thorough physical examination is conducted. This includes a series of assessments designed to rule out other potential causes of the symptoms the patient is experiencing. Through this meticulous process, healthcare providers can gather essential information that aids in diagnosing and formulating a suitable treatment plan.

2. **Gastric Emptying Study (GES)**

    The Gastric Emptying Study stands as the cornerstone diagnostic test for gastroparesis. During this procedure, the patient consumes a specially prepared meal laced with a safe radioactive marker. Following the ingestion of this meal, a series of scans are conducted at various intervals over a span of several hours.

These scans are critical as they meticulously track the progression of the food as it makes its way through the stomach. The primary indicator for gastroparesis is observed when there is a noticeable delay in the stomach's ability to empty its contents.

This delay, captured through the scans, provides definitive evidence supporting a diagnosis of gastroparesis, enabling healthcare professionals to tailor an appropriate treatment plan.

3. Upper Gastrointestinal (GI) Endoscopy

Widely referred to as an esophagogastroduodenoscopy (EGD), this advanced medical procedure empowers physicians to closely examine the upper portion of the digestive system. By utilizing a flexible, slender tube outfitted with a light and camera at its tip, doctors can navigate through the esophagus, stomach, and beginning of the small intestine (duodenum) with precision.

This technique is pivotal in diagnosing by allowing direct visualization of the inner lining of these organs, hence identifying any potential blockages, ulcers, inflammation, tumors, or other abnormalities that could be the root cause of various symptoms. The insights gained from an EGD are invaluable in formulating an effective treatment plan for the patient.

4. Upper GI Series or Barium X-ray

This diagnostic procedure requires the patient to drink a special liquid containing barium. This substance is noteworthy for its ability to coat the lining of the upper gastrointestinal (GI) tract, which includes the stomach, esophagus, and small intestine. Once the barium has been ingested, a series of X-rays are taken.

These X-rays provide exceptionally clear images of the upper GI tract, allowing physicians to easily identify any abnormalities or issues present. The detailed views afforded by this method make it an invaluable tool in diagnosing a range of conditions affecting these parts of the digestive system.

5. Blood Tests

These are crucial diagnostic tools that play a significant role in the medical field. They are designed to check for a wide range of underlying health issues, including but not limited to diabetes, thyroid disorders, or other potential conditions that may be contributing to the patient's symptoms.

Through the analysis of various components of the blood, such as red and white blood cell counts, glucose levels, and hormone concentrations, healthcare providers can gain valuable insights into the patient's overall health status.

This information allows them to pinpoint specific issues that need to be addressed and develop a targeted treatment plan. By understanding the detailed makeup of the blood, doctors can make informed decisions about patient care, leading to better health outcomes and more personalized medicine.

6. **SmartPill**

This innovative diagnostic tool represents a significant advancement in gastrointestinal health monitoring. By swallowing a small, capsule-sized device, patients enable doctors to measure vital parameters such as pH levels, temperature, and pressure throughout the digestive tract.

This sophisticated technology can shed light on the digestive process by providing detailed information on the transit time of food through the system, offering valuable insights into various conditions that might affect digestion. It's a non-invasive method that promises to revolutionize the diagnosis and management of gastrointestinal disorders.

7. **Electrogastrography (EGG)**

   While not as widely utilized as other techniques, EGG is a diagnostic test that records the electrical activity of the stomach to evaluate its motility. By placing electrodes on the patient's body, it captures the stomach's electrical signals.

   An abnormal EGG pattern can indicate issues like gastroparesis, a condition where the stomach takes too long to empty its contents, potentially leading to a variety of symptoms and affecting overall digestive health.

The diagnosis of gastroparesis is typically considered once other potential causes for the symptoms have been excluded. It's important to accurately diagnose gastroparesis to ensure appropriate management and treatment strategies are employed, as symptoms can closely resemble those of other gastrointestinal disorders.

Medical Treatments of Gastroparesis

Medical treatments for gastroparesis focus on managing symptoms and promoting gastric emptying. The approaches can vary based on the severity of the condition and underlying causes. Common treatments include:

Dietary Changes

Adopting a diet consisting of small, frequent meals that are low in both fat and fiber can significantly ease digestive symptoms. For individuals who have difficulty with solid foods, liquid or pureed foods may be recommended due to their ease of digestion. This dietary adjustment can help in managing symptoms and improving overall digestive health.

Medications to Stimulate Stomach Muscles

Medications like Metoclopramide (Reglan) are specifically designed to increase the contractions of the stomach, facilitating the process of stomach emptying and aiding in the digestion of foods more efficiently.

Besides promoting the movement of food, Metoclopramide also plays a crucial role in reducing the occurrences of nausea and vomiting. Erythromycin, which is traditionally used as an antibiotic, has been found to have a similar effect on the stomach, stimulating the emptying process and contributing to a smoother digestive process.

Medications to Control Nausea and Vomiting

To manage and control the discomforting symptoms of nausea and vomiting, healthcare providers often recommend antiemetics such as ondansetron (Zofran) or promethazine (Phenergan). These medications are effective in calming the stomach and providing relief from these frequent and uncomfortable symptoms, making the overall condition more manageable for the patient.

Gastric Electrical Stimulation

In more severe cases where standard treatments do not provide adequate relief, a gastric neurostimulator, commonly referred to as a "gastric pacemaker," may be surgically implanted. This innovative device is designed to send mild, carefully regulated electrical pulses to the stomach muscles, which helps in controlling nausea and vomiting by enhancing the stomach's natural motility.

Jejunostomy Tube

For patients facing severe cases where oral nutrition is not sufficient or possible, a more direct method of nutritional support may be implemented through the placement of a jejunostomy tube. This feeding tube is inserted directly into the small intestine, bypassing the stomach entirely, to ensure that the patient receives the necessary nutrients for survival and recovery without exacerbating their condition.

Parenteral Nutrition

In the most extreme cases, where oral or enteral nutrition is not feasible, parenteral nutrition becomes a critical life saving intervention. Through this method, a comprehensive blend of nutrients is delivered directly into the bloodstream via an intravenous (IV) line.

This approach ensures that the patient's nutritional needs are met, even when the digestive system is not functional, allowing for the provision of essential vitamins, minerals, and calories necessary for the body's functioning and recovery process.

The choice of treatment depends on the severity of the gastroparesis, its underlying cause, and how it has responded to previous treatments. A multidisciplinary approach, often involving dietitians, gastroenterologists, and sometimes surgeons, is crucial for effective management.

Lifestyle Changes to Manage the Gastroparesis

Managing gastroparesis often involves a combination of medical treatments, lifestyle adjustments, and natural remedies. These strategies aim to alleviate symptoms, improve gastric emptying, and enhance quality of life. Here are some recommended changes to manage the gastroparesis;

- *Eat Smaller, More Frequent Meals:* Consuming smaller volumes more frequently can help manage symptoms by reducing the workload on the stomach.
- *Chew Food Thoroughly*: Chewing food well can aid in digestion and make it easier for the stomach to process.
- *Limit High-Fiber Foods*: Foods high in fiber, such as raw fruits and vegetables, can be harder to digest and

should be consumed in moderation. Cooking or pureeing these foods can make them easier to digest.
- *Avoid High-Fat Foods*: Fatty foods slow down gastric emptying. Opt for low-fat options when possible.
- *Stay Hydrated*: Drinking non-carbonated, low-fat, and preferably clear liquids throughout the day can help with hydration without aggravating symptoms.
- *Avoid Lying Down After Meals*: Remaining upright for at least two hours after eating can help with gastric emptying.
- *Monitor Blood Sugar Levels*: For those with diabetes, controlling blood sugar levels can prevent further damage to the vagus nerve.

Natural Remedies for Gastroparesis

Aside from lifestyle changes, there are also natural remedies that can help manage gastroparesis symptoms. These include:

- *Ginger*: Known for its gastrointestinal benefits, ginger can help alleviate nausea and improve gastric motility. It can be consumed as tea, in food, or as a supplement.
- *Acupuncture*: Some people find relief from gastroparesis symptoms with acupuncture, a traditional Chinese medicine technique that involves inserting thin needles into specific points on the body.
- *Probiotics*: These beneficial bacteria can help maintain gut health. Although research on probiotics for

gastroparesis is limited, they may aid in overall digestive health.

- ***Peppermint Oil***: Some evidence suggests peppermint oil can help relax the muscles of the gastrointestinal tract, potentially improving symptoms. However, it should be used cautiously, as it can also relax the sphincter between the stomach and esophagus, leading to worsen GERD symptoms.

It's essential to consult with a healthcare provider before making significant dietary changes or adding supplements to your regimen, especially if you have underlying health conditions or are taking medications. Personalized advice from a dietitian or a specialist in gastroenterology can be invaluable in managing gastroparesis.

Gastroparesis and Women

Recent statistics show that about 80% of idiopathic cases of gastroparesis are experienced by women. In one report, there was even a notable rise of cases in young women since 2014. Usually, these cases are either divided among those with diabetes or are considered idiopathic. However, for those young women who are being diagnosed with gastroparesis, their condition is usually related to autoimmune diseases, such as lupus, rheumatoid arthritis, and thyroid disease. Also, it was noted that usually, these young women are overweight.

According to experts, women are more prone to be diagnosed with gastroparesis than men. Women's stomach motility is slower compared to men's due to the possibility of having higher levels of female sex hormones and nitric oxide, according to one study.

Symptoms are also more prevalent, and even severe, in women than in men. Usually, patients feel sick after eating—they experience nausea, stomach pain, vomiting, and bloating. Even when they eat only a small amount of food, they already feel full and feel like they eat too much.

According to Dr. Michael Cline of Cleveland Clinic, usually, when food in the stomach isn't digested, it's pushed out through vomiting.

Until now, it's still unclear why there's a significant difference between men and women who suffer from this condition. However, there is still something that can be done to treat it and relieve the patients from the symptoms.

What Is Gastroparesis Diet?

A gastroparesis diet is a dietary plan designed specifically for patients with gastroparesis. It involves choosing foods that are easy to digest and avoiding those that can aggravate the symptoms of the condition.

The main goal of this diet is to help regulate and improve the patient's digestion, minimizing the discomfort and severity of their symptoms. In the next section, we will discuss the principles, benefits, and potential drawbacks of a gastroparesis diet.

The gastroparesis diet is tailored to minimize symptoms and support nutritional needs by adapting how and what you eat. The key principles include:

1. ***Eat Small, Frequent Meals***: Large meals can overwhelm a slow-emptying stomach. Eating smaller amounts more frequently can help manage symptoms and ensure nutrient intake is spread throughout the day.
2. ***Choose Low-Fiber Foods***: Fiber slows down digestion and can form bezoars (indigestible material) in the stomach, exacerbating symptoms. Limit high-fiber

foods like raw fruits and vegetables, whole grains, and legumes.

3. ***Limit Fats***: Fat naturally slows stomach emptying. Opt for low-fat foods to ease digestion. However, incorporating small amounts of healthy fats is important for overall nutrition.

4. ***Stay Hydrated***: Drink plenty of fluids throughout the day. Opt for non-carbonated and sugar-free options where possible. Sometimes, liquid meal replacements are suggested for their ease of digestion and nutrient content.

5. ***Chew Food Well***: This makes it easier for your stomach to process food and can aid in symptom management.

6. ***Avoid Tough Meats and Fibrous Fruits and Vegetables***: These can be difficult to digest. Choosing cooked fruits and vegetables over raw ones and tender cuts of meat can help.

7. ***Consider Liquid Nutrition***: For some, solid foods are too difficult to digest. Smoothies, soups, and other liquid-based foods can provide necessary nutrients while being easier on the stomach.

8. ***Monitor Your Tolerance***: Different people have different tolerances to foods. Keeping a food diary can help identify which foods trigger symptoms and which are well-tolerated.

9. ***Gradually Increase Dietary Fiber***: In some cases, once symptoms improve, slowly adding soluble fiber back into the diet can help with overall gastrointestinal health. This should be done carefully and under the guidance of a healthcare provider.
10. ***Consult a Dietitian***: Ideally, work with a dietitian experienced in managing gastroparesis. They can help develop a personalized eating plan that meets your nutritional needs and lifestyle.

Implementing these dietary principles can significantly help manage gastroparesis symptoms and improve quality of life. Each person's response to certain foods can vary, so it's important to adjust the diet based on personal tolerance and nutritional needs.

Benefits of the Gastroparesis Diet

Adopting a gastroparesis diet can offer several benefits for individuals dealing with this challenging condition. By adjusting eating habits to accommodate the stomach's delayed emptying, patients can experience improvements in both symptoms and overall well-being. Key benefits include:

1. ***Reduced Symptoms***: The primary goal of the gastroparesis diet is to minimize common symptoms such as nausea, vomiting, bloating, and abdominal pain. Smaller, more frequent meals and the avoidance

of hard-to-digest foods can significantly alleviate these discomforts.
2. *Improved Nutrient Absorption*: By selecting foods that are easier to digest, this diet helps ensure that the body can better absorb essential nutrients, which might otherwise be difficult due to impaired gastric function.
3. *Enhanced Gastric Emptying*: Low-fat and low-fiber foods can facilitate smoother and quicker stomach emptying, reducing the risks of complications such as bezoars (indigestible masses) and bacterial overgrowth from undigested food.
4. *Better Blood Sugar Control*: For people with diabetes and gastroparesis, managing carbohydrate intake through the diet can help prevent spikes and drops in blood sugar levels, contributing to overall glucose control.
5. *Increased Energy Levels*: By improving nutrient intake and digestion, individuals may experience boosts in energy and decreased fatigue, as the body is better nourished.
6. *Weight Management*: Effective management of gastroparesis through diet can also help maintain a healthy weight by preventing malnutrition or unintentional weight loss, a common issue in those with severe symptoms.
7. *Personalized Nutrition*: Working with a dietitian to tailor the gastroparesis diet to individual needs allows

for a balanced intake of vitamins, minerals, and other nutrients, ensuring that dietary restrictions do not lead to deficiencies.
8. **Enhanced Quality of Life**: By reducing the severity of gastroparesis symptoms and improving overall nutritional status, individuals can enjoy a better quality of life with fewer disruptions from their condition.

Incorporating the principles of the gastroparesis diet requires thought, planning, and sometimes creativity, but the potential benefits for symptom management and nutritional health make it a critical component of living with gastroparesis.

Potential Drawbacks

While the gastroparesis diet offers significant benefits to those suffering from this condition, like any specialized diet, it comes with its potential drawbacks. However, it's important to note that for most individuals with gastroparesis, the benefits of following this diet significantly outweigh these disadvantages.

1. **Limited Food Variety**: The need to avoid high-fiber and high-fat foods can make the diet seem restrictive, potentially leading to mealtime monotony. This limitation can affect enjoyment of meals and social eating situations.
2. **Nutritional Deficiencies**: The diet's restrictions can also make it harder to get a full range of nutrients. For

example, limiting fiber intake might impact digestive health, while avoiding certain fruits and vegetables can reduce antioxidant intake.
3. **Social and Emotional Impact**: Dining out or eating at social events can be challenging, leading to feelings of isolation or frustration. It might require more planning and communication about dietary needs.
4. **Initial Symptom Management**: It may take time to see improvements in symptoms, and finding the right balance of foods that are tolerable can be a process of trial and error, which might be discouraging for some.
5. **Weight Management Issues**: For some, ensuring adequate calorie intake on this diet can be difficult, potentially leading to weight loss or malnutrition. Others may find managing weight harder due to the limitations on food choices.

By understanding these potential drawbacks, individuals can prepare for and manage them accordingly. For example, seeking support from a registered dietitian who specializes in gastroparesis diets can help address nutritional concerns.

5 Step-by-Step Guide to Getting Started with the Gastroparesis Diet

Starting a gastroparesis diet can seem daunting at first, but it's a manageable process when you follow these carefully outlined steps. This diet aims to minimize your symptoms and ensure you're still getting the nutrition you need. Here's how you can get started:

Step 1: Familiarize Yourself with Gastroparesis

Gaining a comprehensive understanding of gastroparesis is the foundational step in managing its impact on your life. Gastroparesis, also known as delayed gastric emptying, is a medical condition where the stomach's muscle movements are slowed down or don't work at all, preventing your stomach from emptying properly. This disruption can lead to a range of uncomfortable and sometimes debilitating symptoms.

The primary symptoms of gastroparesis include nausea and vomiting, which can become particularly severe after eating.

Many people with this condition also experience a feeling of fullness shortly after starting a meal, even if they've eaten only a small amount.

This early satiety can make it challenging to consume enough calories and nutrients, leading to weight loss and malnutrition over time. Bloating is another common symptom, often accompanied by abdominal pain, which can range from mild discomfort to severe pain that interferes with daily activities.

Understanding how gastroparesis affects your body goes beyond recognizing symptoms. It involves learning about the potential causes of the condition, such as diabetes, surgical interventions in the abdominal area, viral infections, or idiopathic reasons where no cause can be identified. Knowing the underlying cause can sometimes help tailor treatment and management strategies more effectively.

Understanding gastroparesis and its impact on digestion is crucial. Normally, food moves through the digestive tract thanks to strong muscle contractions. With gastroparesis, these contractions are weak or absent, causing food to stay in the stomach longer, which can lead to bacterial overgrowth from food fermentation. Additionally, food can form hard masses called bezoars that block the path to the small intestine.

By grasping gastroparesis's effects, you can make informed choices about your diet, lifestyle, and care. It helps you identify foods and habits that worsen or improve symptoms. With this knowledge, you can work effectively with healthcare providers to create a treatment plan tailored to your needs. Understanding your condition also means you can explain it to family, friends, and employers, creating a support system for your health management.

Step 2: Shift Towards Liquid Nutrition

Adopting a liquid-based diet is an effective strategy for managing the symptoms of gastroparesis. Given the condition's impact on digestive efficiency, liquids can be a soothing alternative to solid foods, offering nutritional support without placing undue strain on the stomach. Here's how to effectively incorporate liquids into your dietary regimen:

Understanding the Importance of Liquids

Liquids are inherently easier for the stomach to process because they require less gastric motility—the series of muscle contractions that move food through the digestive tract—compared to solids. This characteristic makes liquids particularly beneficial for individuals with gastroparesis, as it can help mitigate common symptoms like nausea and vomiting, and reduce the feeling of fullness and bloating after eating.

Selecting the Right Liquids

Not all liquids are created equal, especially when it comes to managing a sensitive condition like gastroparesis. It's crucial to choose drinks that provide nutritional value while being gentle on the digestive system:

- *Clear Broths*: Rich in vitamins and minerals, clear broths are soothing, easy to consume, and provide hydration. Opt for low-fat and low-sodium versions to avoid aggravating your symptoms.
- *Herbal Teas*: Herbal teas, such as ginger or peppermint tea, can offer calming effects on the digestive system. They are also caffeine-free, ensuring they don't stimulate gastric acidity or lead to dehydration.
- *Nutrient-Rich Smoothies*: Smoothies made by blending well-tolerated fruits and vegetables can be an excellent way to receive essential nutrients. Incorporate protein powders or Greek yogurt to increase the protein content, but be mindful to blend thoroughly to a smooth consistency and avoid high-fiber ingredients that can be difficult to digest.

Monitoring Your Body's Response

Each person's experience with gastroparesis is unique, making it vital to observe how your body reacts to different types of liquids. Some may find certain herbal teas more soothing than others, while some might prefer the consistency or nutritional profile of specific smoothies. Tracking your reactions can guide you to make informed adjustments, optimizing your liquid diet to suit your personal tolerances and preferences.

The Role of Hydration

Staying adequately hydrated is paramount for overall health, and even more so for individuals with gastroparesis. Dehydration can exacerbate symptoms and contribute to further complications. Apart from consuming broths and teas, ensure you're drinking plenty of water throughout the day. Sometimes, electrolyte solutions or rehydration salts may be necessary to maintain electrolyte balance, especially if vomiting is a frequent symptom.

Gradual Introduction and Adjustment

Transitioning to a liquid nutrition plan should be approached gradually, giving your body time to adjust. Starting with one liquid meal a day and progressively increasing as tolerated can help ease the transition. Always consult with a healthcare provider or a dietitian specializing in gastroparesis to ensure your nutritional needs are met during this adjustment phase.

By focusing on liquid nutrition, you're taking an important step in managing gastroparesis, allowing your digestive system to rest while ensuring you remain nourished and hydrated. Remember, this approach is typically temporary or part of a broader management plan, including solid foods as your condition permits.

Step 3: Introduce Low-Fiber Solids Gradually

Transitioning from a liquid-based diet to incorporating solid foods is a significant step in managing gastroparesis. This phase aims to carefully reintroduce your digestive system to solids without overwhelming it. Here's how you can smoothly make this transition:

Understanding Low-Fiber Solids

The focus during this stage is on low-fiber solids—foods that are simpler for your stomach to break down and move along. High-fiber foods, while generally healthy, can slow gastric emptying even further in individuals with gastroparesis, leading to increased discomfort. Low-fiber options provide the necessary calories and nutrients with less risk of exacerbating symptoms.

Selecting Digestion-Friendly Foods

Your choice of foods during this phase is crucial. Opt for those that are known for their ease of digestion:

- *Starches*: White bread, white rice, and potatoes (peeled) are excellent sources of energy. They lack the fibrous outer layers found in their whole-grain or skin-on counterparts, making them gentler on your stomach.

- ***Proteins***: Lean proteins such as chicken, turkey, and fish are easier to digest compared to fatty cuts of meat. They offer essential amino acids without putting too much strain on your digestive system.
- ***Vegetables and Fruits***: While many fruits and vegetables are high in fiber, you can still enjoy certain types by cooking them well and removing skins and seeds. Examples include canned peaches or pears (in their own juice, not syrup), boiled carrots, and strained vegetable soups.

Cooking Methods Matter

How you prepare these foods can make a significant difference in how well they're tolerated:

- ***Steaming and Boiling***: These methods are gentle on the food, preserving its nutritional value while making it softer and easier to digest.
- ***Grilling***: Grilling should be done with care to avoid charring the food, which can make it harder to digest. Use foil to wrap the food and retain moisture, making it softer and more palatable.
- ***Avoid Frying***: Frying adds extra fat, which can significantly slow down digestion and aggravate symptoms. Stick to the above methods for a safer alternative.

Gradual Introduction

Start by introducing one low-fiber solid food at a time, observing how your body responds to each addition. If a particular food doesn't cause any adverse effects, you can consider keeping it in your diet and slowly introducing another. This careful, methodical approach allows you to build a personalized diet plan that suits your digestive capabilities.

Listen to Your Body

Paying close attention to your body's signals is paramount. If certain foods trigger symptoms, take note and avoid them moving forward. It's normal to have some trial and error during this process, as gastroparesis affects everyone differently.

Step 4: Carefully Manage Fat and Fiber

Navigating fat and fiber intake is a delicate balancing act in the management of gastroparesis. Both can influence how quickly your stomach empties, affecting your symptoms and overall comfort. Understanding how to manage these dietary components can significantly enhance your quality of life.

The Impact of Fat and Fiber

Fat is known to slow gastric emptying, a process that is already compromised in gastroparesis. High-fat foods can exacerbate symptoms such as nausea and fullness. Similarly, while fiber is beneficial for digestive health in general, it can be problematic for those with gastroparesis because high-fiber foods may be more challenging to digest and can linger in the stomach.

Optimizing Fat Intake

While it's important to moderate your fat intake, completely eliminating fat is not advisable due to its essential role in overall health. Fats are crucial for absorbing certain vitamins and providing energy. Here's how to approach fat in your diet:

- ***Choose Healthy Fats***: Incorporate sources of unsaturated fats, like avocado, nuts, seeds, and olive oil, which offer health benefits without the negative impact of saturated and trans fats found in many processed foods.
- ***Low-Fat Cooking Methods***: Steam, boil, bake, or grill your foods without adding extra fat. If you do use oil, opt for a light spray or a small amount of healthy oil, like olive or canola oil.
- ***Monitor Portions***: Even healthy fats should be consumed in moderation. Small, frequent meals with controlled fat content can help manage your symptoms more effectively.

Managing Fiber Intake

Fiber's role in a gastroparesis diet can be complex. While it's a critical component of a healthy diet, it may worsen symptoms for some individuals with gastroparesis. To incorporate fiber safely:

- *Limit High-Fiber Foods*: Initially, reduce the intake of raw fruits and vegetables, whole grains, legumes, and seeds until you understand how your body responds to fiber.
- *Blend or Puree Foods*: High-fiber foods can sometimes be made more digestible by blending or pureeing them. This can include making smooth soups from vegetables or creating fruit smoothies.
- *Introduce Fiber Gradually*: Start with low-fiber options and slowly introduce more fibrous foods one at a time. Pay attention to your body's response and adjust accordingly.

Strategies for Implementation

- *Keep a Food Diary*: Documenting your fat and fiber intake alongside your symptoms can help identify what works best for you. Note the types of fats and fibers that your stomach handles well.
- *Consult a Dietitian*: A healthcare professional specializing in dietary management can provide personalized advice on balancing fat and fiber with

gastroparesis, ensuring you meet your nutritional needs without exacerbating symptoms.

Step 5: Keep a Detailed Food Diary

Maintaining a detailed food diary is an essential step in managing gastroparesis effectively. This practice involves meticulous record-keeping of your dietary intake and subsequent physical reactions, providing invaluable insights into how different foods and beverages influence your symptoms. Here's how to implement this strategy effectively:

The Importance of a Food Diary

A food diary acts as a personalized guide to understanding your gastroparesis. It can reveal patterns and triggers that may not be immediately apparent, allowing you to make informed adjustments to your diet. The goal is to optimize your nutrition while minimizing discomfort and symptoms.

What to Record

To get the most out of your food diary, include detailed information about:

- *Food and Beverage Intake*: Write down everything you consume, including main meals, snacks, and drinks. Be specific about ingredients in mixed dishes.
- *Symptom Tracking*: Note any symptoms that occur after eating, such as nausea, bloating, pain, or

vomiting. Include the severity and duration of these symptoms.
- ***Portion Sizes***: Quantify your food intake as accurately as possible. Understanding portion sizes can help identify if the volume of food affects your symptoms.
- ***Time of Day***: Record the time you eat and experience symptoms. This can help identify if symptom patterns are related to meal timing.
- ***Emotional State***: Stress and emotions can significantly affect digestive processes. Note your emotional state before and after meals to see if there's a correlation between stress and symptom flare-ups.

Analyzing Your Diary

Regularly reviewing your food diary is a critical step in managing symptoms of digestive disorders, such as gastroparesis. This diary isn't just a log of what you eat; it's a powerful tool for uncovering specific patterns and connections between your dietary habits and the symptoms you experience. Over time, this detailed record can reveal insights that are crucial for adjusting your diet to better suit your body's needs.

When analyzing your food diary, start by looking for any clear correlations between certain foods or eating behaviors and the onset or worsening of symptoms. This might include noting how quickly after eating particular foods your symptoms appear, as well as their severity and duration. For instance, you might find that high-fiber foods lead to more severe bloating and discomfort, or that eating large meals exacerbates nausea and delays gastric emptying.

It's also important to pay attention to the timing of your meals and symptoms. Gastroparesis requires careful management of not just what you eat, but when you eat. Smaller, more frequent meals might result in fewer symptoms than three larger meals a day. Through your food diary analysis, you might discover that symptoms are less pronounced earlier in the day, suggesting that your largest meal should be at breakfast rather than dinner.

In addition to identifying trigger foods and problematic eating patterns, your food diary can help you pinpoint foods that you tolerate well. These "safe foods" can form the foundation of your gastroparesis-friendly diet. By focusing on these foods, you can maintain nutritional balance and variety in your diet, which is essential for overall health and well-being.

Analyzing your diary should be an ongoing process. The effectiveness of dietary changes can vary over time due to fluctuations in your condition or other factors, such as stress or medication changes. Regularly revisiting your diary helps adapt your diet to these changes, ensuring that your management strategy remains effective.

Furthermore, sharing your food diary with healthcare professionals can provide them with valuable insights into your condition. A dietitian or nutritionist can use this information to offer personalized advice, helping you to further refine your diet and manage your symptoms more effectively. They can suggest substitutions for eliminated foods, ensuring that you do not miss out on essential nutrients.

In essence, your food diary is much more than a log; it's a guide that helps you and your healthcare team make informed decisions about your diet. By continually analyzing and adjusting based on your diary, you can develop a diet that minimizes your symptoms, supports your nutritional needs, and improves your quality of life.

Sharing Your Findings

Your food diary is not just a personal resource but also a tool for communication with healthcare professionals. Sharing your diary with your doctor or dietitian can provide them with a deeper understanding of your condition. They can use this information to offer more tailored advice, potentially adjusting medications or suggesting specific dietary interventions based on your documented experiences.

Tips for Effective Diary Keeping

- ***Stay Consistent***: Aim to write in your diary every day. Consistency is key to creating a useful record of your experiences. Think of your diary as a daily ritual, something that is as much a part of your routine as brushing your teeth or having breakfast. The more regularly you update it, the more valuable a resource it will become, offering insights into your habits and patterns over time.

- *Be Honest*: It's absolutely vital that you record all information as truthfully as possible, especially when it comes to keeping a food diary. If you indulge in foods that might not be the best for your health or your condition, it's important to note that down. Honesty in your diary ensures you have a clear picture of your lifestyle, which is crucial for making any positive changes.
- *Use Technology*: In today's digital age, consider leveraging technology to aid your diary-keeping practices. There are numerous smartphone apps available designed specifically for food tracking. These apps often come with added features that allow you to also track symptoms, moods, and emotions, providing a more comprehensive view of your health. Using an app can make the process of keeping a diary much more convenient and user-friendly, allowing you to make entries on the go and have all your information in one easily accessible place.

Adapting to the gastroparesis diet is a personal and ongoing process. It requires patience, experimentation, and close attention to how your body reacts to different foods. Work closely with your healthcare provider to ensure your diet remains nutritionally balanced while effectively managing your symptoms.

Foods to Include in the Gastroparesis Diet

When managing gastroparesis, selecting the right foods to include in your diet is crucial for minimizing symptoms and ensuring nutritional intake. Here's a list of foods generally recommended:

Low-Fiber Vegetables

- Cooked vegetables: carrots, spinach, mushrooms, potatoes (without skin)
- Vegetable juices (without pulp)

Lean Proteins

- Chicken (skinless and white meat)
- Turkey (skinless and white meat)
- Fish and shellfish
- Egg whites or well-cooked eggs
- Low-fat cuts of pork or beef chewed thoroughly

Refined Grains

- White bread, pasta, and rice
- Low-fiber cereals
- Crackers and pretzels made from refined flour

Fruits

- Canned or cooked fruits without skins or seeds (e.g., applesauce, canned peaches or pears)
- Banana (ripe and well-mashed)
- Fruit juices without pulp

Dairy

- Low-fat or fat-free milk and yogurt (for those who can tolerate lactose)
- Small amounts of cheese, preferably low-fat

Soups and Broths

- Clear broths and soups with well-cooked or pureed vegetables and lean proteins

Beverages

- Water (plain or flavored without carbonation)
- Herbal teas (non-caffeinated)
- Nutritional supplement drinks (consult with a dietitian for suitable options)

Others

- Small amounts of smooth nut butter (like almond or peanut butter)
- Honey and syrups (in moderation)

Foods to Eat with Caution (might be tolerated by some)
- Avocado (in small amounts, as it's higher in fat but also provides beneficial nutrients)
- Soft, scrambled eggs or omelets (ensure they are well-cooked)

It's important to personalize your diet based on what you can tolerate. Some individuals may find they can handle certain foods that others cannot. Starting with easily digestible foods and gradually introducing new items while monitoring symptoms can help identify what works best for you.

Foods to Avoid in the Gastroparesis Diet

Managing gastroparesis often requires avoiding foods that can exacerbate symptoms due to their difficulty in digesting or their propensity to delay gastric emptying further. Here's a list of foods generally recommended to avoid or limit:

High-Fiber Foods
- Raw fruits and vegetables, especially those with skins and seeds
- Legumes such as beans, lentils, chickpeas
- Whole grains and bran products
- Tough, fibrous meats (e.g., steak)
- Dried fruits and fruit with membranes (e.g., oranges, grapefruits)

High-Fat Foods

- Fried foods and greasy foods
- Full-fat dairy products
- Fatty meats (e.g., sausage, bacon, ribs)
- Fast food
- Rich pastries, doughnuts, and other high-fat baked goods

Certain Vegetables and Fruits

- Cruciferous vegetables like broccoli, cauliflower, cabbage, and Brussels sprouts due to their high fiber content
- Corn, including popcorn, because of its difficult-to-digest hulls

Others

- Nuts and seeds, including foods containing whole seeds
- Carbonated beverages, as they can produce gas and bloat
- Chewing gum and hard candies, as they can increase the intake of air, leading to bloating
- Alcohol and caffeine (in coffee, tea, some soft drinks, and chocolate), as they can stimulate the stomach and irritate the digestive system

It's crucial to work with a healthcare provider or dietitian when managing gastroparesis. They can offer personalized advice and adjustments to ensure your nutritional needs are met while avoiding triggers for your symptoms. Balancing a restrictive diet with adequate nutrition is key to managing gastroparesis effectively.

Here's a more organized sample meal plan tailored for the gastroparesis diet. Remember, the key is to consume small, frequent meals and steer clear of foods that may trigger symptoms.

Sample Meal Plan for the Gastroparesis Diet

Following a gastroparesis diet doesn't mean you can't enjoy delicious and nutritious meals. This sample meal plan includes options for breakfast, lunch, dinner, and snacks that are suitable for those with gastroparesis.

Day 1

Breakfast: Fruit Smoothie

AM Snack: Rice cake with peanut butter and jelly

Lunch: Chicken Seafood Paella

Noon Snack: Celery sticks with cream cheese

Dinner: Blended Soup

PM Snack: Puréed fruit salad (apples, grapes, bananas)

Day 2

Breakfast: Muesli-Style Oatmeal

AM Snack: Lemon-Vanilla Berry Parfaits

Lunch: Vegetable Stir-Fry with Cauliflower Rice

Noon Snack: Celery sticks with cream cheese

Dinner: Chicken and Broccoli over Cauliflower Rice

PM Snack Puréed fruit salad (apples, grapes, bananas)

Day 3

Breakfast: Mango Honey Green Smoothie

AM Snack: Almond Surf Smoothie

Lunch: Grilled Chicken Kebabs

Noon Snack: Celery sticks with cream cheese

PM Dinner: Turkey with Avocado Salad

PM Snack: Puréed fruit salad (apples, grapes, bananas)

Day 4

Breakfast: Broccoli and Cheese Omelet

AM Snack: Celery sticks with cream cheese

Noon Lunch: Lentil Soup

Noon Snack: Rice cake with peanut butter and jelly

Dinner: Avocado and Salmon Salad

PM Snack: Fruit Smoothie

Day 5

Breakfast: Greek Yogurt Parfait with Berries and Almonds

AM Snack: Rice cake with peanut butter and jelly

Lunch: Turkey and Avocado Salad

Snack: Almond Surf Smoothie

Dinner: Guilt-Free Egg Salad

PM Snack: Celery sticks with cream cheese

Day 6

Breakfast: Muesli-Style Oatmeal

AM Snack: Rice cake with peanut butter and jelly

Lunch: Honey Roasted Potatoes

Snack: Lemon-Vanilla Berry Parfaits

Dinner: Grilled Chicken Kebabs

PM Snack: Almond Surf Smoothie

Day 7

Breakfast: Lentil Soup

AM Snack: Almond Surf Smoothie

Lunch: Chicken Seafood Paella

Snack: Celery sticks with cream cheese

Dinner: Asian Zucchini Salad

PM Snack: Puréed fruit salad (apples, grapes, bananas)

Coping with Gastroparesis

Living with gastroparesis presents a unique set of challenges, as the symptoms can drastically impact day-to-day life. However, adopting effective coping strategies can significantly enhance your quality of life and symptom management.

Essential Tips for Managing Gastroparesis

- ***Seek Support***: Actively connect with support groups, both online and in person. These groups can provide emotional encouragement and practical tips from individuals who truly understand what you're going through. Sharing experiences and strategies can be incredibly helpful.
- ***Educate Yourself***: Deepen your understanding of gastroparesis. The more comprehensive your knowledge about the condition, the better equipped you'll be to manage its complexities. Being well-informed allows you to make decisions about your care that are best suited to your needs.

- ***Build a Care Team***: Work closely with healthcare professionals who have a deep understanding of gastroparesis. Having a dedicated and knowledgeable team is crucial for the development of an effective treatment plan. This team should be flexible, and ready to adjust your plan as your condition changes over time.
- ***Exercise Patience***: The journey of managing a chronic condition like gastroparesis is long and requires both time and patience. It's important to be kind to yourself and acknowledge the small victories along the way. Progress can be slow, but every step forward counts.
- ***Implement Lifestyle Adjustments***: Make dietary and lifestyle changes to significantly alleviate symptoms of gastroparesis, thereby enhancing your overall well-being. This could include modifying the consistency of your food, eating smaller, more frequent meals, and identifying foods that trigger symptoms to avoid them.
- ***Explore Alternative Therapies***: Beyond traditional medical treatments, consider exploring alternative therapies such as acupuncture or hypnotherapy. These methods may offer additional relief from symptoms for some individuals. It's important to consult with your care team to ensure these therapies complement your existing treatment plan effectively.

Troubleshooting the Gastroparesis Diet

If adhering to the gastroparesis diet proves challenging, the following tips may help refine your approach:

- *Prioritize Small, Frequent Meals*: Instead of three large meals, aim for smaller, more frequent meals throughout the day. This approach can significantly ease the digestive strain by not overwhelming your stomach.
- *Identify and Avoid Trigger Foods*: Pay close attention to how your body reacts to different foods. Document these reactions and work to eliminate any foods that consistently cause discomfort or exacerbate your symptoms. This can be a crucial step in managing your condition effectively.
- *Stay Hydrated*: Drinking enough fluids, especially water, is vital not only for digestion but for overall bodily functions. Adequate hydration helps in the smooth processing of nutrients and the elimination of wastes.
- *Opt for Soft, Bland Foods*: Incorporating foods that are easy to digest and low in spices and fats can help prevent an aggravation of symptoms. Soft, bland foods tend to be less irritating to the stomach lining.
- *Ensure Nutritional Balance*: Given the dietary restrictions that may come with managing your condition, it might be challenging to get all the

necessary nutrients from food alone. Supplements could play a key role in ensuring you receive a balanced spectrum of nutrients.

- *Maintain a Food Diary*: By keeping a detailed record of what you eat and how it affects you, you can gain insights into which foods are beneficial and which are problematic. This diary can be an invaluable tool for customizing your diet to minimize symptoms.
- *Collaborate with Healthcare Professionals*: Building a relationship with doctors and dietitians who understand gastroparesis can provide you with personalized advice and support. This professional guidance is crucial for effective management of the condition.
- *Be Patient with Progress*: Understanding that adjustments in diet and lifestyle may not yield immediate results is important. Patience and persistence in following your treatment plan, while continuously evaluating and adjusting it with the help of healthcare professionals, are key to finding what works best for you.

By integrating these strategies, individuals living with gastroparesis can achieve better symptom control and an improved quality of life.

Sample Recipes

Below are some recipes that are safe for the gastroparesis diet. Remember to avoid trigger foods and to eat small, frequent meals.

Blended Soup

Ingredients:

- 1 cup puréed vegetables
- 1 cup chicken or vegetable broth
- 1/2 cup cooked rice, pasta, or beans
- 1/4 cup milk or cream
- salt
- pepper

Instructions:

1. In a pot, combine puréed vegetables and broth over medium heat.
2. Add in cooked rice, pasta or beans and stir until heated through.
3. Stir in milk or cream and season with salt and pepper to taste.
4. Remove from heat and let cool before blending until smooth.
5. Reheat before serving if necessary.

Fruit Smoothie

Ingredients:

- 1 cup puréed fruit
- 1 cup milk or yogurt
- 1/2 cup ice

Instructions:

1. Combine all ingredients in a blender.
2. Blend until smooth and frothy.
3. Serve immediately.

Vegetable Stir-Fry

Ingredients:

- 1 cup vegetables, puréed
- 1/2 cup cooked rice, pasta, or beans
- 1 tbsp. olive oil
- salt
- pepper

Instructions:

1. Heat the oil in a pan over medium heat.
2. Add the puréed vegetables and cook for 5 minutes.
3. Add the rice, pasta, or beans and cook for 5 more minutes.
4. Season with salt and pepper to taste.
5. Serve with crackers or bread.

Asian Zucchini Salad

Ingredients:

- 1 medium zucchini, sliced thinly into spirals
- 1/3 cup rice vinegar
- 3/4 cup avocado oil
- 1 cup sunflower seeds, shells removed
- 1 lb. cabbage, shredded
- 1 tsp. stevia drops
- 1 cup almonds, sliced

Instructions:

1. Cut the zucchini spirals into smaller parts. Set aside.
2. Put almonds, sunflower seeds, and cabbage in a large bowl. Combine the ingredients well.
3. Add zucchini to the mixture.
4. In a small bowl, mix vinegar, stevia, and oil using a whisk or fork.
5. Pour the vinegar mixture all over the zucchini mixture. Toss well. Make sure everything is covered with the dressing.
6. Refrigerate for 2 hours before serving.

Honey Roasted Potatoes

Ingredients:

- 2 lb. cubed red potatoes
- 2 tbsp. honey
- 2 tbsp. olive oil
- 1/2 tsp. crushed rosemary
- 1 tsp. salt
- 1 tsp. mustard powder
- pepper, to taste

Instructions:

1. Set the oven to 375 °F.
2. Make the honey mixture by mixing honey, olive oil, salt, pepper, rosemary, and mustard powder in a small bowl.
3. Spray some nonstick spray on the baking pan.
4. Put potatoes in the pan and mix with the honey mixture. Place in the preheated oven and cook for about 35 minutes.

Guilt-Free Egg Salad

Ingredients:

- 125 ml. mayonnaise, full-fat variety
- 6 eggs, hard-boiled
- some fresh parsley, chopped
- 1 tsp. curry powder, or to taste

Instructions:

1. Peel the hard-boiled eggs and chop them into small pieces.
2. In a large bowl, mix together mayonnaise, curry powder, and chopped parsley.
3. Add the chopped eggs to the mixture and combine well.
4. Serve chilled on top of bread or crackers or as a side dish for a main meal.

Turkey with Avocado Salad

Ingredients:

- 1 lb. lean ground turkey
- 1 avocado, sliced
- 1 can of black olives
- 2 heads romaine lettuce, hand rip to bite-sized pieces
- 2 tbsp. extra-virgin olive oil
- 1 tsp. balsamic vinegar
- 1/2 tsp. sea salt

Instructions:

1. Heat a skillet over medium heat and add the ground turkey. Cook until browned, stirring occasionally.
2. In a small bowl, mix together olive oil, balsamic vinegar, and sea salt to make the dressing.
3. In a large salad bowl, combine lettuce, sliced avocado, and black olives.
4. Add cooked ground turkey on top of the salad.
5. Drizzle the dressing over the salad and toss to combine.
6. Serve as a healthy and filling lunch or dinner option.

Cauliflower Rice with Chicken and Broccoli

Ingredients:

- 1 broccoli head
- 1 cauliflower head
- 2 chicken breasts, boneless and skinless
- 1 tbsp. olive oil
- salt
- pepper

Instructions:

1. Preheat the oven to 375°F (190°C).
2. Cut the broccoli and cauliflower into bite-sized pieces.
3. Place the chicken breasts in a baking dish and season with salt and pepper.
4. In a separate bowl, mix together broccoli, cauliflower, olive oil, salt, and pepper.
5. Spread the mixture around the chicken breasts in the baking dish.
6. Bake for 25-30 minutes, or until chicken is fully cooked and vegetables are tender.
7. Serve as a delicious low-carb alternative to traditional rice dishes.

Lentil Soup

Ingredients:

- 1 tbsp. avocado oil
- 1 cup onion, diced
- 1/2 cup carrot, diced
- 1/2 cup celery, diced
- 4 cups vegetable or chicken broth
- 1 cup dried red lentils, well rinsed
- 1/4 tsp dried thyme
- 1/2 cup fresh flat-leaf parsley, chopped
- salt
- pepper

Instructions:

1. Sauté carrot, celery, and onion in a large saucepan over medium heat. Do so until they are soft.
2. Pour in the broth, with lentils and thyme, and wait for it to boil.
3. Lower the heat. Cover and leave to simmer until lentils are soft, about 20 minutes.
4. Transfer soup into a blender.
5. Set the blender on high. Purée the soup until it's creamy.
6. If it's too thick, pour in a cup of water.

7. Add salt and pepper, to taste.
8. Return to the saucepan to reheat if necessary.
9. Ladle into bowls and garnish with parsley.
10. Serve and enjoy while hot.

Greek Yogurt Parfait with Berries and Almonds

Ingredients:

- 1 cup Greek yogurt
- 1 cup mixed berries
- 1/4 cup almonds, chopped
- 2 tbsp. honey

Instructions:

1. In a small bowl, mix together Greek yogurt and honey.
2. In a separate bowl, combine berries and almonds.
3. Layer half of the yogurt mixture into two glasses or bowls.
4. Add half of the berry and almond mixture on top of the yogurt layer.
5. Repeat layers with the remaining ingredients.
6. Serve as a healthy and tasty breakfast or snack option.

Muesli-Style Oatmeal

Ingredients:

- 1/2 banana, diced
- 1 cup instant oatmeal
- 1/2 golden apple, peeled and diced
- 1 cup milk
- 2 tbsp. raisins
- 2 tsp. honey or sugar
- a pinch of salt

Instructions:

1. In a bowl, mix oatmeal, raisins, milk, sugar or honey, and salt.
2. Put on a cover and refrigerate.
3. Leave the mixture overnight or for at least 2 hours.
4. Get it out of the fridge after the allotted time then serve with fruits.
5. Add some milk if the mixture gets too thick.
6. Serve while warm.

Broccoli and Cheese Omelet

Ingredients:

- 1 egg
- 2 egg whites
- 1 tbsp. skim milk
- salt
- fresh pepper
- oil spray
- 1/2 cup broccoli, cooked
- 1 slice WW reduced fat 1 pt Swiss cheese

Instructions:

1. Beat together egg and egg whites. Add in milk and season with pepper and salt according to taste.
2. Place a non-stick skillet on medium heat.
3. Lightly spray the pan with oil.
4. Carefully add the scrambled eggs into the pan, covering it completely. Lower the heat.
5. Place the cheese in the center. Add the broccoli on top.
6. Once the eggs are set, flip over the sides to the center.
7. Serve and enjoy while warm.

Almond Surf Smoothie

Ingredients:

- 1 large banana
- 1 tbsp. almond butter
- 1 cup almond milk
- 1/8 tsp. vanilla extract
- 1 tbsp. wheat germ
- 1/8 tsp. ground cinnamon
- 3–4 ice cubes

Instructions:

1. In a blender, add the banana, almond butter, almond milk, vanilla extract, wheat germ, and cinnamon.
2. Blend until smooth.
3. Add in the ice cubes and blend again until the desired consistency is reached.
4. Pour into a glass and serve immediately.
5. Optional: top with sliced almonds for added crunch and protein.

Mango Honey Green Smoothie

Ingredients:

- 2 pcs. bananas
- A handful of large spinach
- 1 pc. mango, sliced
- 1 tbsp. honey
- 3-4 pcs. ice cubes

Instructions:

1. In a blender, add the bananas, spinach, mango slices, and honey.
2. Blend until smooth.
3. Add in 3-4 ice cubes and blend again until desired consistency is reached.
4. Pour into a glass and serve immediately.
5. Optional: top with additional mango slices for added flavor and texture.

Lemon-Vanilla Berry Parfaits

Ingredients:

- 1 cup low-fat yogurt
- 2 tbsp. honey
- 2 containers of fat-free vanilla pudding
- 1 lemon zest
- 2 tbsp. lemon curd
- fresh mint leaves
- 1 tbsp. fresh lemon juice
- 1/2 tsp. vanilla extract
- 3 cups mixed berries, such as strawberries, raspberries, and blueberries

Instructions:

1. Whisk together the pudding, yogurt, vanilla extract, and lemon curd in a small bowl. Set aside.
2. Mix lemon zest, lemon juice, and honey in another mixing bowl. Stir well until fully combined.
3. Add in the mixed berries. Use a rubber spatula to gently stir to coat.
4. Assemble the parfaits in four 8-ounce glasses.

5. Scoop three tablespoons of the yogurt mixture into each glass. Top them with 1/4 cup of mixed berries. Repeat the process to have two 6. layers of the yogurt mixture and berries.
6. Garnish each parfait with fresh mint and cover.
7. Refrigerate for a couple of hours.
8. Serve and enjoy while chilled.

Avocado and Salmon Salad

Ingredients:

- 1/4 avocado, peeled with pit discarded
- 1 tbsp. lemon juice
- 2 tsp. extra-virgin olive oil
- 1 tsp. Dijon mustard
- salt
- black pepper, freshly ground
- 4 oz. canned wild salmon, with bones, no salt added
- 2 tbsp. celery, sliced
- 2 tbsp. parsley, finely chopped

Instructions:

1. In a medium bowl, combine the avocado, lemon juice, olive oil, mustard, salt, and pepper.
2. Mash the avocado with the back of a fork, and combine thoroughly with the other ingredients.
3. Flake the salmon, and add it to the avocado mixture.
4. Add the celery and parsley.
5. Serve immediately.

Grilled Chicken Kebabs

Ingredients:

- 1 tbsp. garlic, minced
- 1/2 tsp. Himalayan pink salt, fine
- 1/2 tsp. black pepper, freshly ground
- 2 tsp. fresh oregano, minced, or 1 tsp. dried oregano
- 1 tbsp. extra-virgin olive oil
- 1 tbsp. lime juice, freshly squeezed
- 1-1/2 lb. chicken breast, boneless and skinless

Instructions:

1. In a small bowl, combine the garlic, salt, black pepper, oregano, olive oil, and lime juice.
2. Cut the chicken breast into bite-sized cubes and add them to the marinade.
3. Toss well to coat all pieces evenly with the marinade.
4. Cover and refrigerate for at least an hour or overnight.
5. Soak wooden skewers in water for at least 30 minutes to prevent them from burning on the grill.
6. Preheat your grill to medium-high heat.
7. Thread the chicken pieces onto the skewers, leaving a small space between each piece to ensure even cooking.

8. Grill for about 10-12 minutes, turning occasionally, until the chicken is cooked through and slightly charred on the edges.
9. Serve hot with your choice of sides such as grilled vegetables or a salad.

Chicken Seafood Paella

Ingredients:

- 6 chicken thighs, skinless
- 3 cups Arborio rice
- 6 pcs. each of the seafood ingredients: mussels, scallops, and clams of choice
- 2 ham hocks
- 2 cups seafood stock
- 4 tbsp. cooking oil, divided
- 1 cup carrots, chopped roughly
- 1 cup red bell pepper, diced
- 1 cup celery, roughly chopped
- 1 lb. Mexican style chorizo
- 1 cup apple cider vinegar
- 1 tbsp. saffron mixed with 1 cup water, steeped for 3 minutes
- salt
- black pepper
- 1/2 cup scallions, diced, for garnish

Instructions:

1. Pour 2 tablespoons of oil into a large stockpot placed over high heat.
2. Add ham hocks and chicken and cook until both thighs are evenly brown on each side.
3. Transfer chicken to a plate and set aside.

4. Continue cooking ham hocks. Add carrots and celery. Sauté for 7 minutes.
5. Deglaze by pouring white wine then decrease by half.
6. Pour seafood stock, around 2 quarts of water, and saffron mixture. Simmer to reduce liquid by half for 2 hours.
7. Once done, strain the broth and simmer over low heat.
8. Heat the remaining oil in a paella pan.
9. Sauté chorizo, remaining onion slices, and red bell pepper. Cook until translucent without browning onions.
10. Add rice and season with salt and freshly ground black pepper according to preference.
11. Stir until rice grains are coated with oil.
12. Set rice around the pan to level then pour a cup of stock at a time without stirring.
13. Check if the rice is al dente or almost fully cooked then add the seafood ingredients and chicken thigh.
14. Cover seafood with rice to cook. Add the last cup of broth then cover the pan tightly.
15. Remove from heat and let paella sit for 15 minutes or until newly added ingredients are cooked.
16. Serve and enjoy while hot.

Creamy Mashed Potatoes

Ingredients:

- 2 large potatoes, peeled and cubed
- 2 tablespoons butter (or a low-fat alternative)
- 1/4 cup low-fat milk or almond milk
- Salt to taste

Instructions:

1. In a pot, add the peeled and cubed potatoes and enough water to cover them.
2. Bring the water to a boil and let the potatoes cook for about 15 minutes or until they are soft when pierced with a fork.
3. Drain the water from the potatoes and return them to the pot.
4. Mash the potatoes using a potato masher or fork until they are smooth.
5. Add the butter and mix until fully incorporated.
6. Gradually add in the milk, stirring until desired consistency is reached.
7. Season with salt according to taste.
8. Serve hot as a side dish or use as a topping for shepherd's pie or other dishes.
9. For a creamier texture, you can also add in some cream cheese or sour cream.

Poached Pears in Cinnamon Syrup

Ingredients:

- 4 ripe pears, peeled, halved, and cored
- 4 cups water
- 1/2 cup sugar
- 2 cinnamon sticks
- A dash of vanilla extract

Instructions:

1. In a saucepan, combine water, sugar, cinnamon sticks, and vanilla extract. Bring to a boil.
2. Add the pear halves and reduce the heat to a gentle simmer.
3. Let pears cook for about 10 minutes or until they are fork-tender.
4. Remove pears from the syrup and let them cool before serving.
5. Optional: Reduce the syrup until it thickens and serve alongside poached pears as a topping. This light and naturally sweet dessert is an easy way to satisfy a sweet tooth without causing discomfort for those with gastroparesis. Plus, it's packed with fiber and nutrients from the pears!

Silken Tofu with Soy Sauce and Scallions

Ingredients:

- 1 block silken tofu, drained
- 2 tablespoons low-sodium soy sauce
- 1 scallion, finely chopped (optional)
- A sprinkle of sesame seeds

Instructions:

1. Cut the tofu into cubes and place on a microwave-safe plate.
2. Microwave for 1-2 minutes, or until heated through.
3. Drizzle with soy sauce and top with scallions and sesame seeds.
4. Enjoy as a light meal or snack, packed with protein and easily digestible. You can also add some cooked rice to make it more filling.

Simple Baked Apples

Ingredients:

- 4 apples, cored
- 2 tablespoons brown sugar
- 1/2 teaspoon cinnamon
- 1/4 cup water

Instructions:

1. Preheat the oven to 375°F.
2. In a small bowl, mix together brown sugar and cinnamon.
3. Place the cored apples on a baking dish and sprinkle with the sugar-cinnamon mixture.
4. Add water to the bottom of the dish and bake for about 30 minutes, until tender.
5. Serve warm with a dollop of whipped cream or vanilla ice cream for a comforting and gentle dessert. Baked apples are also a good source of fiber, which can help with digestion and promote regular bowel movements.

Quinoa Porridge

Ingredients:

- 1 cup quinoa, rinsed
- 2 cups low-fat milk or a milk alternative
- 2 tablespoons maple syrup
- 1/2 teaspoon vanilla extract
- Fresh berries for topping (optional)

Instructions:

1. Combine quinoa and milk in a saucepan and bring to a boil.
2. Reduce heat to low, cover, and simmer until most of the milk is absorbed and the quinoa is tender, about 15 minutes.
3. Stir in maple syrup and vanilla extract.
4. Serve topped with fresh berries if desired. This porridge is a more nutrient-dense alternative to traditional grains, offering a higher protein content which is beneficial for maintaining energy levels.

Each recipe in this collection has been designed to be gentle on the digestive system while providing nutritional value and variety, catering to the needs of individuals managing gastroparesis.

Conclusion

Congratulations and thank you for taking the time to complete this comprehensive guide on the gastroparesis diet. By now, you've embarked on a valuable journey toward understanding and managing gastroparesis through dietary modifications that cater specifically to your body's needs. It's a significant step forward in enhancing your quality of life and gaining control over your symptoms.

The path to managing gastroparesis is highly personal and can be challenging, but remember, you're not alone in this. Armed with the knowledge from this guide, you're now equipped to make informed decisions about what to eat, how to prepare your meals and the best ways to consume them to alleviate your symptoms. The strategies and tips provided here are designed to help you maintain nutrition, avoid discomfort, and enjoy a variety of foods despite the limitations that gastroparesis imposes.

One of the key insights from this guide is the importance of listening to your body. Everyone's experience with gastroparesis is unique, and what works for one person may not work for another. Pay close attention to how different foods affect you, and adjust your diet accordingly. It may be helpful to keep a food diary to track your meals and symptoms, allowing you to identify patterns and make necessary adjustments more effectively.

It's also crucial to focus on small, manageable changes. Overhauling your diet overnight can be overwhelming and unsustainable. Instead, take it one step at a time. Start by introducing low-fiber, low-fat foods that are easier to digest, and gradually build up from there. Remember, small progress is still progress.

Staying hydrated is another vital component of managing gastroparesis. Drinking enough fluids is essential for digestion, but remember to sip slowly throughout the day rather than consuming large amounts at once. This can help prevent feelings of fullness and nausea.

In addition to dietary changes, remember to consult regularly with your healthcare provider. They can offer personalized advice, support, and adjustments to your treatment plan as needed. Your dietitian or nutritionist can also be an invaluable resource in helping you adapt your diet to meet your nutritional needs without exacerbating your symptoms.

Remember, managing gastroparesis is a marathon, not a sprint. There will be good days and bad days, but each step you take toward understanding and adapting your diet brings you closer to better health and well-being. Be patient with yourself and recognize the effort you're putting in. Celebrate the small victories, like finding a new recipe that works for you or going a day without major symptoms.

If you find yourself feeling frustrated or overwhelmed, reach out for support. Whether it's friends, family, healthcare professionals, or online communities, having a support network can make all the difference. Sharing your experiences, challenges, and successes with others who understand can be incredibly comforting and empowering.

Finally, never lose sight of the fact that your diet is just one piece of the puzzle when it comes to managing gastroparesis. A holistic approach that includes stress management, physical activity as tolerated, and medication or treatments recommended by your healthcare provider can provide the best outcomes.

Thank you once again for dedicating your time and energy to learning from this gastroparesis diet guide. We hope it serves as a valuable tool in your journey towards better health. Remember, every step forward, no matter how small, is a victory in managing your symptoms and leading a fuller, more enjoyable life. Stay encouraged, stay informed, and most importantly, stay hopeful. You've got this!

FAQs

What foods should I avoid if I have gastroparesis?

Avoid high-fiber foods such as whole grains, raw fruits and vegetables, nuts, and seeds, as they can slow down stomach emptying. Also, reduce intake of fatty foods, including fried foods, full-fat dairy products, and fatty cuts of meat, which can exacerbate symptoms.

Can I still eat fruits and vegetables if I have gastroparesis?

Yes, but you may need to modify how you consume them. Cooked, canned, or pureed fruits and vegetables are easier to digest. Always remove skins and seeds, and opt for low-fiber varieties like canned peaches or green beans.

How often should I eat if I have gastroparesis?

Eating small, frequent meals can help manage symptoms. Aim for 4-6 smaller meals throughout the day rather than three large ones to prevent overloading your stomach.

Is it okay to drink fluids during meals?

It's usually recommended to limit fluid intake during meals to avoid feeling too full. Try to drink fluids between meals instead. However, everyone is different, so monitor how your body responds and adjust accordingly.

How can I ensure I'm getting enough nutrients on a gastroparesis diet?

Since the gastroparesis diet limits certain foods, consider working with a dietitian to ensure you're meeting your nutritional needs. Supplements may be necessary for some individuals to compensate for the restrictions.

Are there any specific cooking methods that are recommended for the gastroparesis diet?

Gentle cooking methods like steaming, boiling, baking, and grilling are recommended. These methods can make food easier to digest by preserving its nutritional value while making it softer.

What should I do if my symptoms flare up despite following the gastroparesis diet?

Flare-ups can still occur due to stress, illness, or other factors unrelated to diet. Keep a detailed food diary to identify any potential triggers or patterns. If flare-ups become frequent or severe, consult your healthcare provider for further evaluation and management.

References and Helpful Links

Wiginton, K. (2024, March 17). Is there a gastroparesis diet? WebMD. https://www.webmd.com/digestive-disorders/gastroparesis-digestive-disorders

Gastroparesis - NIDDK. (n.d.). National Institute of Diabetes and Digestive and Kidney Diseases. https://www.niddk.nih.gov/health-information/digestive-diseases/gastroparesis#:~:text=Gastroparesis%2C%20also%20called%20delayed%20gastric,in%20the%20stomach%20or%20intestines.

Professional, C. C. M. (n.d.-c). Gastroparesis. Cleveland Clinic. https://my.clevelandclinic.org/health/diseases/15522-gastroparesis

Whnp-Bc, L. S. M. B. (2023a, June 20). Gastroparesis: What you need to know. https://www.medicalnewstoday.com/articles/313873

Leonard, J. (2023, May 18). Best foods and diet tips for gastroparesis, and what to avoid. https://www.medicalnewstoday.com/articles/318753

Mbbs, K. K. (2022, July 8). Gastroparesis Diet: Foods to Avoid, Foods to Eat & Diet Plan. MedicineNet. https://www.medicinenet.com/gastroparesis_diet_foods_to_avoid_foods_to_eat/article.htm

www.ingramcontent.com/pod-product-compliance
Lightning Source LLC
LaVergne TN
LVHW012032060526
838201LV00061B/4568